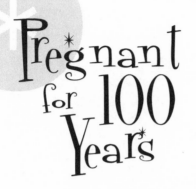

From conception
to contractions . . .
Real moms tell all!

Pregnant for 100 Years

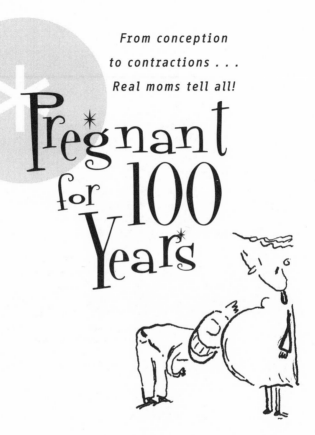

Jeanne Benedict

A Perigee Book

A Perigee Book
Published by The Berkley Publishing Group
A division of Penguin Group (USA) Inc.
375 Hudson Street
New York, New York 10014

Copyright © 2004 by Jeanne Benedict
Cover design and illustration by Laura Cornell
Package design by Dorothy Wachtenheim
Text design by Tiffany Estreicher

Perigee hardcover edition: April 2004

Visit our website at www.penguin.com

Library of Congress Cataloging-in-Publication Data

Benedict, Jeanne.
    Pregnant for 100 years : from conception to contractions . . . : real moms tell
all / Jeanne Benedict.
        p.   cm.
    ISBN 0-399-52967-5
    1. Pregnancy—Anecdotes.   2. Pregnancy—Popular works.   I. Title.

RG525.B455   2004
618.2—dc22

                                                        2003065932

Printed in the United States of America

10   9   8   7   6   5   4   3   2   1

For John, Dylan, and Piper

Contents

Acknowledgments

To all the mothers, fathers, siblings-to-be, family members, and birth pros who shared their best prenatal quotes, labor stories, and nostalgic pregnancy tales, thank you.

For John Duff, I thank you for a friendship that has far too many miles between it and for the times when we do enjoy each other's company in person, be it over an elegant dinner or in the sky-high cafeteria where you point across the Hudson River to remind me where I was born in case I get too uppity. Thanks to Sheila Curry Oakes, whose wit and smarts make her a great editor and new friend.

A lot of love to my glamorous pregnant girlfriends Justine Reiss and Raye Dowell, who flank me in the media companion video for this book and who are totally honest about which maternity clothes make you look fabulous and the outfits that make you look like freight. Thanks to all who immediately granted the big "woman with child" a favor because she really looked like she needed one, including Wexler Video, Set Stuff, Mom's the Word, Mezzomondo, Ralph's Grocery Store, Marie et Cie., John Sparano, Shane Rogers, Elise Bruccoliere, Kristin Eichle the yoga goddess and the yoga ladies, Lori Dorman at the Birth Connection, East Valley Family YMCA and its delightful members, Dr. Lloyd Greig, Dr. Barry Brock, Rosie Flores, Dr. Tsui, Bob Benedict, Chris Jackson, Erin and Vaughn Neimiec, Charlienne Barnes, Eliot Markman, Dan Benedict, Wendy Worthington, Kelly Conway, and, most of all, Dylan, Reese, Hannah, Gussie, and Willa.

As always, my heart melts each time my husband, John, and son, Dylan, walk into a room, play wrestle, pick flowers for me, and have a kiss at the ready simply because I'm there. I am so very lucky that we share this life of laughter and love. Thank you for being the family of my dreams.

And finally to Piper, the little girl in my womb whom we are all so excited to meet in six weeks and who is kicking me as I write this, reminding me that it was she who sparked many of the inspirations reflected in this book.

Introduction

O ne never knows what hysterical, hormonal words will come out of the mouth of a pregnant woman, especially when in the company of veteran moms. And then the stories of childbirth, morning sickness, weight gain, big kicks, and little bumps swell like a belly on that special nine-month mission. It's like we can't help ourselves. The idea for this book was born from one of those contagious conception-and-beyond conversations at a baby shower.

I was newly pregnant, about five weeks along, and not telling anyone . . . until I got into a roomful of women at a baby shower. Something about the stack of stuffed animals on the gift table and the big pink bow on the deluxe stroller made me blurt out, "I'm pregnant too!" as I hugged my expectant friend, the guest of honor. I took my seat at the table and the usual questions came my way—"When are you due?" and "Do you know what you are having?" Yes, I knew my due date and the only thing I knew I *wasn't* having at this brunch event was the champagne.

Across the table was this elegant woman, in her sixties I would guess, who just happened to own this upscale Malibu restaurant that we were dining at. As she spoke, I discovered that she had quite the real estate portfolio, including a little piece of a Hawaiian island, and often lectured on business matters at a prestigious university. When the customary "baby talk" began, this very powerful woman shared her delivery experience: "My doctor didn't believe in any pain medication. So, naturally, when in labor I was screaming my head off. The doctor looked up at me and said, 'For God's sake, Anne, would you shut up!' and I was silent throughout the birth." I was floored and fascinated. How far we've come in this process from the early 1960s, when the conventional birthing method was the old knock-'em-out and drag-'em-out, to the present-day ritual of the proud father cutting the cord.

Then the younger women at the table chimed in—"When I was pregnant my breasts were so big I felt like I was carrying three babies!" and from the end of the table a joke: "Hey, do you know what they call London socialites who opt for a scheduled C-section?" "What?" we all shouted back. "Too posh to push!" I didn't know if this conversation was more appropriate for a women's locker room or a quilting bee. But I did know that it would make an entertaining book.

My hope is that every pregnant woman who reads this book finds a little gem, a word of wisdom, or even a good comeback line to use on those strangers lacking in prenatal etiquette who feel they can approach you and say anything to you. Also, I wanted to keep the entries short and sweet, geared toward the clock of the pregnant bladder. Pick it up, have a chuckle, shed a tear, head for the potty, and repeat. My wish is that *Pregnant for 100 Years* offers up a little something for all, with just enough sass for the bonbon girls and just enough sentimentality for those who cherish every little kick from within.

Chapter One

To Dream the In Utero Dream

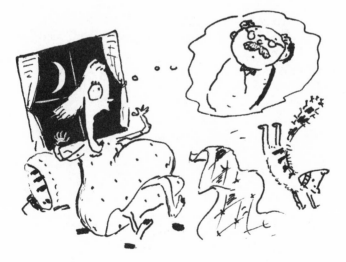

"My baby was such a fierce womb kicker that one night I dreamt a dragon popped out of my belly."

- **Evelyn, attorney, pregnant 1989, 1992**

✳

"Toward the end of my pregnancy both the baby and I were getting really restless. I had this dream that I was wrestling an alligator poolside. We fell into the water and relaxed."

- **Tori, travel agent, pregnant 1975, 1978, 1980**

"I had this dream that my baby extended her hand while inside my womb with her impression visible through my skin and shook hands with me."

- **Marie, book editor, pregnant 2001**

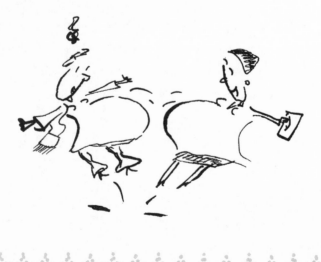

"At eight months pregnant I had an ultrasound to check on the size of the baby. Actually I was more interested to see what in the world she was doing in there. It felt like she was performing backflips, and in her ultrasound image she appeared to be bobbing up and down in the womb. That night I dreamt I gave birth to a seal."

• Sarah, secretary, pregnant 1995, 1997

"My husband and I were watching TV when all of a sudden he jumped up and said, 'I had a dream about the baby last night, only she wasn't a baby. She was about seventeen with blonde hair and really sweet. We were invited to a party and she wanted to come along. I remember looking at her in my dream and thinking . . . does she have a beer? And then I realized that she wasn't old enough to drink. She was so lovely and absolutely beautiful. We had done a great job as parents.' At that point I was sobbing."

- Janet, hotel executive, pregnant 1998, 2003

"I dreamt last night that I was giving birth to my baby, and the baby was instructing me on what to do. He was saying things like, 'Don't push now or you'll squeeze my head,' and 'O.K., I'm ready. On your mark, get set, go!' It was so surreal. After he came out he thanked me for a job well done."

• Chris, grocery store manager, pregnant 2003

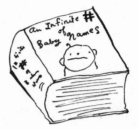

"I had such anxiety about how to take care of a tiny newborn that I dreamt that the baby came out and was like a mini adult. He told me how he'd like to be treated but that I was the one in charge. The dream made me feel like we were in it together and we'd figure it out as we went along."

- **Donna, mom, pregnant 1996, 1999**

"We've been going round and round about names for our baby boy, and of course *everyone* has to give their opinion. It's our own fault because we asked them, but then they have to give you all the variations of nicknames that will torment your child on the playground. In the Jewish faith, it is common to name a child with the first letter of his name starting with the first letter of a deceased relative's name. My uncle Elliot had recently passed away and so we knew that we wanted a baby name starting with *E*. We talked about everything from Edward to Elijah, but still nothing felt quite right. Last night I dreamt that we named the baby Eskimo. He was lying in a white bassinet with this furry hood around his face. I told my husband, and we couldn't stop laughing. We decided to 'chill out' on the baby naming until he arrived and finally decided on Evan."

• **Barbara, owner of a public relations firm, pregnant 2003**

"My baby shower was coming up and my sister, the party queen, had planned this fabulous themed bash. I was really excited about it and wanted so badly to talk about the event but she kept all the little details to herself. I couldn't stand it so I sneaked into her room and peeked at some of the décor. It was a Mexican fiesta! She had painted maracas pink and blue and had adorned these sombreros with pink ribbon. It was so cute! I rushed home and told my husband, who scolded me! I felt so guilty that I had spoiled my own surprise. That night I dreamt that I was at the shower and went into labor. Everyone was around me as I was pushing. But instead of the baby coming out of me there was a loud pop above my head and the baby burst out of a piñata."

• Delia, bookkeeper, pregnant 2001

"I dreamt that my husband was inside the womb with the baby playing patty-cake. All I could think of was that now I'd be taking care of two babies, as my hubby is a big kid at heart."

- **Joy, political fund-raiser, pregnant 2003**

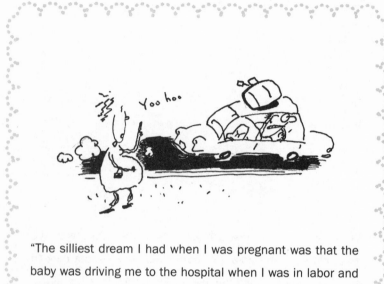

"The silliest dream I had when I was pregnant was that the baby was driving me to the hospital when I was in labor and we got lost."

- **Helen, salesperson, pregnant 1970, 1975, 1978**

"My mother-in-law is always talking about how my husband's brother spoils their children. Well, we are expecting our first baby girl and I fear my husband is going to spoil her rotten just like Veruca Salt. Remember the girl from *Charlie and the Chocolate Factory* whose Daddy gave her everything she wanted and she ended up going down a giant chute? That's Veruca. I had a dream that our baby girl wanted a playhouse and my husband built her a pink castle in the backyard that was bigger than our house. Then my mother-in-law appeared in the dream and asked how we ever expected to pay the mortgage on a big castle. My husband said, 'Relax, Mom, it's made out of candy. Have a gumdrop.' And he corked her mouth with it. I guess the lesson I learned was that he was going to do what he wanted and he didn't care what his mother thought so I shouldn't either. And our nieces and nephews are kind and generous children, spoiled or not."

• Sheila, paralegal, pregnant 2003

"This is weird. My husband dreamt that he was pregnant. He said that I waited on him hand and foot—ironic since he's such a sound sleeper that I've been getting up to fulfill my own midnight cravings. But when he was in the delivery room I was nowhere to be found! He panicked, screaming, 'I can't do this! I don't have the right equipment!' The dream was like a wake-up call (no pun intended) for him to get with the program and pamper his pregnant wife no matter what time it was!"

• **Desiree, store manager, pregnant 1999**

"I had the most wonderful dream when I was pregnant. I was walking through a garden full of baby flowers. Yellow daffodils were beautiful blonde babies with chubby cheeks. Red roses were redheaded babies with a rosy complexion. Brunette babies, oddly enough, were irises. I picked a gorgeous bouquet of the baby flowers and put it in this grand basket on wheels. Then I proceeded up a walkway to an English cottage, where my husband stood in the doorway with a warm, welcoming smile on his face."

- Estella, painter, pregnant 1997, 2000

Chapter Two

The Business of Birthin' Babies

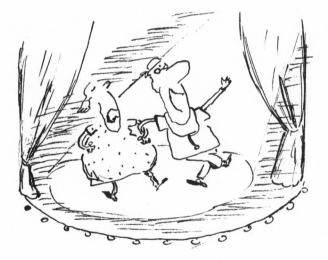

"My doctor didn't believe in any pain medication. So, naturally, when in labor I was screaming my head off. The doctor looked up at me and said, 'For God's sake, Anne, would you shut up!' and I was silent throughout the birth."

• Anne, real estate developer, pregnant 1962

✳

"My doctor induced me a week before my due date because he didn't want to miss his Memorial Day vacation."

• Jane, computer salesperson, pregnant 1963, 1964, 1965, 1969

"On one of my last visits to my OB/GYN before giving birth, I asked her if it was possible to start an I.V. drip of the epidural three or four days before my due date. I was terrified that I wouldn't get one fast enough. What I didn't realize was that I was going to need much stronger drugs to get through the first three months of motherhood, and now that my child is five, I wonder if there is even a drug strong enough to calm me and help me deal with being a mother to a daughter!"

- Angie, hairdresser, pregnant 1997

"It amazes me that today in the year 2003, midwifery is still il-legal in certain states. You'd think that the Supreme Court's decision on a woman's right to choose would extend to her choice of the childbirth process itself."

- **Sandra, midwife since 1989**

✳

"Pregnancy is not a disease, it is a condition."

- **Dr. Lloyd Greig, OB/GYN since 1974**

"I went to see my doctor in a panic as I was convinced there was a problem with the baby and needed to hear the heartbeat to ease my mind. He said, 'We have a word for people like you: mothers.'"

• Dr. Barry Brock, OB/GYN since 1981

"I asked my doctor if you feel any pain with the epidural, and his reply was, 'You've got to break a few eggs to make an omelet.' "

• Dr. P. Simpson, OB/GYN since 1985

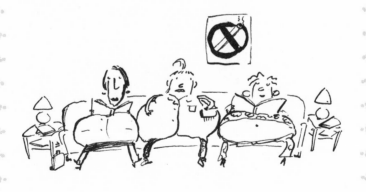

"Seeing your baby in an ultrasound is a miraculous sight! And having the ultrasound technician say, 'This is going to be a pretty baby' is almost amusing. When we asked how she could tell, she replied, 'This baby has a beautiful profile and, believe me, I don't say that to everyone.' We were quite flattered until we overheard her say the same thing to the next couple when they came out of the room."

- **Chandra, lab technician, pregnant 2003**

"I was having horrible pains around six months into my pregnancy. I called my OB/GYN in a panic, thinking that I was going into premature labor. The doctor had me come in immediately for an ultrasound to make sure everything was all right. I was in position on the ultrasound table preparing for the worst. The technician, who was the quiet type, put the glop on my belly and began to scan the baby's image. All of a sudden, she started laughing. I was not amused and blurted out, 'Well, I'm glad you find this funny.' She apologized, turning the monitor so I could see the baby's image, and said, 'No wonder you're in pain. The baby is using your gallbladder as a footrest.'"

• **Annette, video editor, pregnant 2000**

"My wife and I are expecting twins, and she has had a double dose of all pregnancy symptoms. She complained to her doctor, 'Is there anything I can do for the sciatic nerve pain, horrible morning sickness, and migraine headaches?' The doctor said, 'Yes. Give birth.'"

• **Keith, prop house owner, wife pregnant 2000, 2003**

"One of the relaxation exercises in Lamaze class was to close your eyes and go to your happy place. My happy place is what got me there in the first place."

• **Elizabeth, mortgage broker, pregnant 1996, 2000**

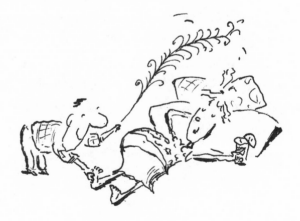

"In my eighth month of pregnancy, my OB/GYN determined that the baby was nearing ten pounds. I started to panic, thinking about how in the world I was going to give birth to a baby that size. 'Is there any way we can stop the baby from growing?' I asked, obviously a bit out of my mind. 'Start smoking,' she replied. *'What?'* I snapped. 'Start smoking,' she repeated, completely deadpan. I had trusted her up to this point and couldn't believe what I was hearing. Oddly enough there was a part of me that took her proposition seriously, thinking maybe that's why babies had much lower birth weights back in the day when no one knew the dangers of smoking while pregnant. 'Start smoking?' I continued, now questioning having her as my doctor. She took a beat and then burst out laughing. Of course she was kidding and I was just glad that my baby was healthy even though he was huge."

- Cynthia, newspaper reporter, pregnant 2001

"We took a Lamaze class just in case we didn't make it to the hospital on time, but I had absolutely no intention of going through birth without pain medication. In class the teacher (who I affectionately called 'Birtha') criticized the hospital that I was delivering at, saying that they gave out epidurals in the parking lot. 'Really? That's great!' I piped up, all cheery, hopeful, and naive. She glared at me and continued showing us how to huff and puff."

• **Celia, gourmet coffee shop owner, pregnant 1997, 2001**

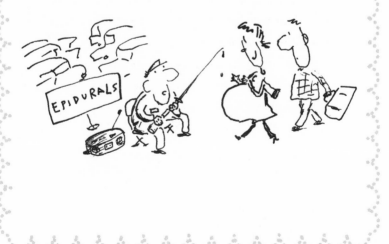

"With the 'he-he-he' and 'ho-ho-ho' breathing that you're sup-posed to do in Lamaze class, all I could visualize was Snow White and the Seven Dwarfs singing, 'Hi ho, hi ho, it's off to work we go. . . . ' I couldn't stop laughing and was asked to leave the room. Outside my husband wanted to know what was so funny. I told him my little joke and he found it amusing as well. We were in labor on the way to the hospital and he began singing, 'Hi ho, hi ho, it's off to birth we go . . . ' Again I cracked up, only this time begged him to stop for fear that my hysterical laughing would push out the baby. I guess the Lamaze class served its purpose."

• Carla, regional sales manager, pregnant 2002

"My friend had to have her baby by C-section but also elected to have a hysterectomy, which was necessary surgery, and a tummy tuck—according to her, even more necessary surgery—at the same time. Where else but in Beverly Hills would a woman have a plastic surgeon tag-team her OB/GYN?"

• Audrey, professional shopper, pregnant 2001

＊

"Although I'm a firm believer in epidurals, I am grateful to those who pushed for natural childbirth in the 1960s. Back then, the motto seemed to be 'knock-'em-out and drag-'em-out.' I couldn't imagine missing the birth of my baby because I was gassed and passed out."

• Mary Ellen, teacher, pregnant 1982, 1984, 1987

Chapter Three

Mothers of Invention

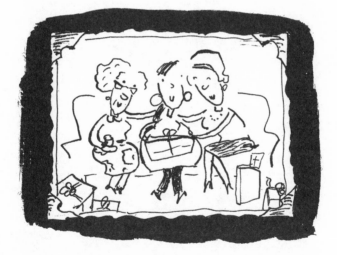

"Fortunately, my grandmother was privileged and could afford chloroform, which was the standard method of pain relief for the upper class during childbirth."

- Martha, speaking of her grandmother, a housewife, pregnant 1901, 1903, 1906

"Having a child or more than one can be such an overwhelming decision. My Irish grandmother had a great saying for those who wanted a larger family but were concerned about money. Her words were, 'You can always put another potato in the pot.'"

- Mandy, speaking of her grandmother, a housewife, pregnant 1944, 1946, 1948, 1950, 1952

"To this very day, my old aunt Pearl believes that excessive reaching or bending can tangle the umbilical cord. Even though I know this falls under the 'old wives' tale' category, I will still ask for someone to pass the salt even if it is right in front of me at the dinner table as opposed to reaching for it like I usually do."

- Jenna, speaking of her aunt Pearl, a seamstress, pregnant in 1932, 1933, 1936, 1938, 1939

"I always wondered why they said 'Boil some water!' when a pregnant pioneer woman went into labor in the movies. I thought it might be for sterilization purposes. Then my great-grandmother told me that they would cut sheets into strips and soak them in the hot water. After they had cooled a bit they would use them as compresses to relieve the pain of labor cramps and contractions."

- Julia, speaking of her great-grandmother, a housewife, pregnant 1918, 1920, 1923, 1924

"My husband was in the military in 1943 when our baby was due. There was a rule that if you had the baby in your hometown you couldn't take off any time, or, as they call it today, maternity leave. So we traveled from Fort Sill, Oklahoma, to a rural part of Iowa where there was no hospital. I gave birth in my mother's living room, and my husband was able to take two weeks off to enjoy his brand-new daughter."

• **Marian, housewife, pregnant 1943**

"My grandmother and I were in the mall shopping for maternity clothes. She saw the store Lane Bryant and suggested we look in there. 'Grandma, I think that store is for larger sized ladies, not pregnant women,' I informed her. I should have known better. Grandma was a retired costume designer and a walking encyclopedia on fashion. Apparently Lane Bryant was the first person to design and sell maternity clothes in 1904 by sewing an elasticized waistband into dresses. 'This was a big deal,' Grandma said. 'Remember, women were still in corsets and many were embarrassed to be seen pregnant in public because they didn't have anything decent to wear. Lane was revolutionary.' As my grandmother spoke, I couldn't imagine being pregnant back then. Just thinking about the added weight of pregnancy and wearing all those long layers of clothes, combined with having to go to the bathroom every fifteen minutes—I never would have left the house either."

- Patricia, speaking of her grandmother, a costume designer, pregnant 1933, 1937

"After having an easy pregnancy resulting in a boy, we decided to do it all again and are expecting a girl. I don't know if it's the stronger connection of the XX that's producing higher hormone levels in my body, but this time around I'm having a much more difficult time. I was at a family gathering, feeling and looking awful as usual, when my old Italian aunt came up to me, patted my pregnant stomach, and said, 'Ah, girls. They steal your beauty.'"

- Marie, speaking of her great-aunt, a bakery owner, pregnant 1942, 1946, 1948, 1950

"Things have sure changed since I had a baby in 1957. Back then they used to conk you out with anesthesia for the birth. I was in labor with my fourth child and had a bad case of the flu. Being a nurse, I knew that problems could develop (like pneumonia) if I was anesthetized with a congested chest. I begged them not to put me under, as I'd been through this three times and could handle it. They didn't listen to me and knocked me out. I got pneumonia and had to wear a surgical mask for a week so the baby didn't catch anything. Worst of all, I couldn't even kiss my baby. Today, that situation would probably result in a lawsuit."

• Selma, nurse, pregnant 1950, 1952, 1954, 1957

"I was doing some research on unassisted home birth and came across the story of a Mrs. Carter in a newspaper article dated 1955. Patricia Carter was a true natural birth pioneer and author of a book entitled *Come Gently, Sweet Lucina.* The newspaper article showed a photo of the lovely Mrs. Carter looking every bit the fifties housewife with a flip hairdo and perfect makeup. However, instead of wearing the classic June Cleaver housedress, she had a large scarf tastefully draped over her nude body as she sat in a chair, apparently ready to give birth to her eighth child. Mrs. Carter's method was to down 'a few whiskey highballs' to relax, excuse herself into the bedroom, take a seat, and catch the baby. She described a brief moment of discomfort, but 'the pain was not nearly as bad as having a tooth pulled.'"

• **Marsha, librarian, pregnant 1964, 1970**

"I called my husband's mom to tell her we were pregnant and the first words out of her mouth were, 'Have you done the Drano test to find out the baby's sex?' This wasn't nearly as bizarre as it sounds, coming from her, as she is a big believer in superstition and old wives' tales. 'Nope,' I said, trying hard not to ask . . . but curiosity got the best of me. 'What is the Drano test?' She went into detail: 'Pee into a glass jar, not plastic, and then when Ben gets home have him mix it with Drano. Don't you mix it because it gives off fumes.' I couldn't resist and put Ben to the task. 'According to your mom,' I giggled, 'if the mixture is greenish brown, green, blue, or has no change it's a girl. Bluish yellow, brownish, or black means boy.' Soon he called his mom and told her, 'I'm standing here with a bluish yellow mixture of pee and Drano.' *'It's a boy!'* I heard her scream over the phone—and he was indeed a boy."

• Claudia, registered dietician, pregnant 1964, 1967

"My mom was on her way to the labor room and the doctor was nowhere to be found. So they parked Mom's gurney off to the side to go find him but I couldn't wait. Mom said she simply pulled up her knees under the blanket and knew I came out when she felt me wiggling between her legs. Later we found out that I was born in the hospital hallway because the doctor went to get a shave."

- **Ethan, mom pregnant 1969, 1971, 1975**

Chapter Four

"About to Pop" Culture

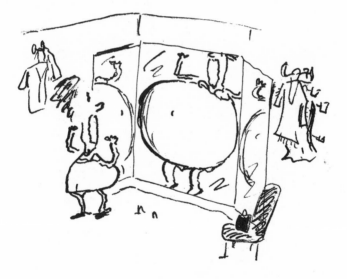

"Before I was pregnant, I gave no thought to tattoo placement. It was only in my eighth month of pregnancy, when the artistic little ink butterfly on my tummy had grown into the Moth That Ate Manhattan, that I questioned my judgment."

• **Melanie, personal trainer, pregnant 2002**

✳

"My mommy girlfriends and I go out for cocktails on Labor Day to celebrate our feats of childbirth."

• **Barrie, attorney, pregnant 1994, 1999**

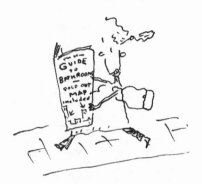

"All my friends flocked to this trendy Los Angeles pregnancy yoga class when they found out they were having a baby. I just couldn't bring myself to sign up. Besides the fact that the whole idea of mantras and group humming gives me the giggles, I could never hold those pretzel positions long enough without having to go pee."

• Nancy, TV producer, pregnant 1998, 2002

"I was complaining about the twenty pounds I had gained during the first and second trimesters of my pregnancy and my Zen girlfriend shut me up by saying, 'The Buddha in me wants to have compassion for you with your weight gain, but if you remember correctly I gained seventy-plus pounds and actually looked like Buddha himself.' "

• Carolina, candle shop owner, pregnant 1996, 1998

"Pregnant women all seem to adopt a certain maternity fashion style. There's 'Sporty Mom,' who usually wears her husband's shirt over leggings and the baseball cap of the moment; 'Goddess Mother,' with a sari draped below her belly and a half shirt letting it all hang out; 'Hippie Mama,' who is a jeans and 1970s, flowing, angel sleeve–top gal; 'Business Mom,' coifed and looking smart, able to efficiently dress for maximum growth with perfectly tailored dark suits and vertical lines; and 'My Baby Mommy,' who wears a lot more pink or blue, depending on if they're having a girl or a boy. Get them all together and you could form a prenatal pop group."

- **Ruth, magazine editor, pregnant 1995, 2000**

"I was so happy to see that maternity clothes go by your prepregnant size. It's like there's a little ray of hope in sight when all you can see is a great big giant belly."

- Wendy, English teacher, pregnant 1994, 1997

"Thank God for those mom friends who give you their maternity clothes the second you announce you're pregnant. Only they know the trauma of seeing your beautiful burgeoning body in the 360-degree view of a dressing room mirror and realizing that you've gone from a size six to a size sixteen."

• Melinda, wardrobe stylist, pregnant 2002

"It's amazing how complete strangers came up to me and touched my pregnant belly without even asking. When this happened to my friend Raye, she would gently put her hand up in defense and say, 'This is sacred space.' I chose to be offensive when this occurred and would yank on their nose or whatever else stuck out on them."

• Nicole, singer, pregnant 1988, 1993

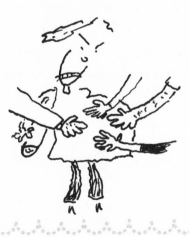

"I was giving an important sales presentation at nine months of pregnancy. All of a sudden the baby started kicking and moving like he was playing rugby. All eyes zeroed in on my stomach except for a few young single guys who averted their eyes and broke out in a sweat, thinking I was going into labor. Well, as the senior ad executive of the firm, I've dealt with more challenging situations. I simply said, 'Seems like the baby is as passionate about this account as I am, and he's willing to fight for it.' Everyone started laughing hysterically. Needless to say we won the client over."

• Emily, senior ad executive, pregnant 2001

"When you are pregnant, alcohol is only for rubbing on sore muscles. But it's sobering, in more ways than the obvious, to realize that, without the benefit of a Cosmopolitan or two, so many of the witty and interesting people you've met at social affairs turn out to be so dull. Either I give too much credit to the alcohol or there's something about pregnancy that lowers your tolerance for bores."

• **Tara, president of a family-owned steel fabricating plant, pregnant 1995, 1998**

"Okay. We all have our hideous stories about having to wear a garish bridesmaid dress. But when you are a pregnant brides-maid you have diplomatic—or undiplomatic—immunity to say whatever you want to protect your image. When my girlfriend showed me the bridesmaid dress she had selected for me to wear in her wedding, I just couldn't keep my mouth shut. My words to her were, 'You know, with the many fluffy layers of ruffles and bows, I fear guests may mistake me for the wed-ding cake.' It was cruel, I know, but the politics of pregnancy can be ruthless."

• Krista, bookstore owner, pregnant 2000

"My good friend Marco is from Mexico, and for Christmas he gave me pink underwear and a pink bra. I thanked him but wasn't sure what to think of such an intimate gift to a pregnant woman. My husband laughed and made a joke about how he always knew that I had an innocent crush on Marco, who happened to be the tall, dark, and handsome type, but to try and seduce a pregnant woman right under the nose of her husband may be just cause for a duel. Well, poor Marco blushed and immediately explained, 'In Mexico, wearing pink underwear on New Year's Day brings the baby good luck.' We thanked him and assured him that we were kidding, but I can see where some husbands may not have appreciated the gift."

- Carrie, hairdresser, pregnant 2002

"When you're pregnant, people in the United States always ask, 'When are you due?' According to my friend from Mexico, when you're expecting, people ask, 'Cuando te alivias?' which basically means 'When do you alleviate yourself?' I think I like the whole idea of being relieved better."

- **Marissa, musician, pregnant 1995**

"I'm a workaholic by nature, but Mother Nature sure takes over when you're pregnant. She makes you tired so you'll rest. She makes you sick so you'll eat the right foods. And she makes the baby in your belly start kicking wildly if you sit and work at the computer for hours on end."

• Penny, Web designer, pregnant 2000, 2003

"I've heard the term 'pregnancy amnesia' used in a couple of ways. Some define the symptom as a state of mind that occurs when you are pregnant, and it's nature's way of letting you forget the little worries like a messy house and helping you to relax so you can concentrate on what's really important—making a baby. And the other definition applies to women about a year or so after pregnancy, and it's where you forget the pain of childbirth so you'll do it all over again."

• **Suzanne, real estate agent, pregnant 1998**

"I've about had it with the pregnancy police. They're the well-meaning, albeit nosy folks who check to make sure that you're drinking decaf as opposed to caffeinated coffee. At grocery stores they trail you, checking out the goods in your cart to make sure you're not going to stuff your face with empty cookie calories as they zero in on your belly and butt to assess your weight gain. They feel compelled to warn you about secondhand smoke, drinking alcohol, and hot Jacuzzis because they have your baby's best interests at heart. I think these self-appointed watchdogs should all be arrested for invasion of privacy."

• Elizabeth, psychologist, pregnant 1992

"Everyone keeps telling me how good I look at six months pregnant. Either they're all big fat liars or I did a great job educating them on what not to say when I was pregnant the first time. Five years ago when pregnant with my son, I got 'Wow, you look great—all big and fat' and 'Don't worry, when you can dye your hair again you'll look a lot younger like you used to.' With this pregnancy I am certainly bigger than I was the first time around and I definitely look and feel more haggard. However, I am dying my hair blonde instead of letting my natural gray roots show under light brown hair. So all I can figure is that they know I'll bite their head off if they say anything except 'You look great' or that blondes appear to have more fun even if they're feeling miserable."

- **Brenda, home accessories designer, pregnant 1997, 2002**

"What is it about a pregnant woman that makes strangers feel as if they can come up to you and say just about anything? They'll tell you all about the harrowing births of their children along with the good and bad labor experiences of friends, loved ones, and anyone they've ever spoken to. I was so sick of it that I started making up stories to retaliate. I told one guy that I was a pregnant mail-order bride and gave him a number where he could get one of his own to start an instant family. I told another woman that I was carrying a 'divine' child, meaning that he was conceived through Immaculate Conception. They kind of look at you like you're crazy and leave you alone. It may sound cruel but now I look forward to meeting new people."

- **Michelle, stand-up comedian, pregnant 2003**

Chapter Five

Hormonal Humor

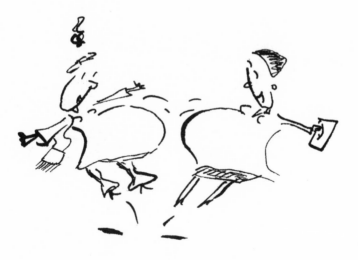

"The difference between birth with an epidural and natural childbirth is the difference between flying first class and flying on the wing."

- Chris, stay-at-home dad, wife pregnant 1998, 2000

"London socialites who opt for a scheduled cesarean section are regarded as 'too posh to push.'"

• Anita, housewife, pregnant 2003

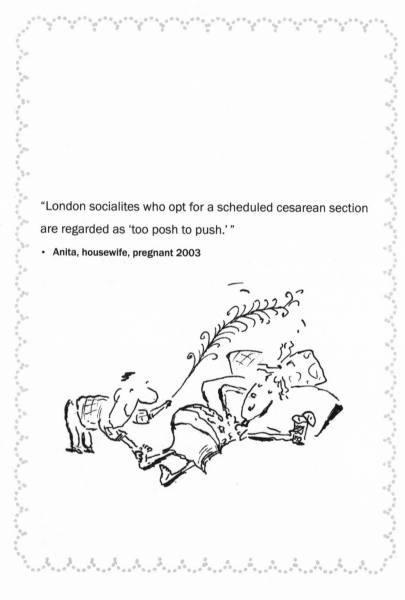

"When I was pregnant I couldn't eat eggs 'cause I felt like I was eating my young."

- Jeanne, author, pregnant 1998, 2003

✳

"It felt like two years that I was pregnant and I was beginning to wonder if I had any relatives who were elephants."

- Carol, X-ray technician, pregnant 1997

"I was so nauseous the other day that I was sure the baby was developing something really important, like a brain."

• Renee, mom, pregnant 2003

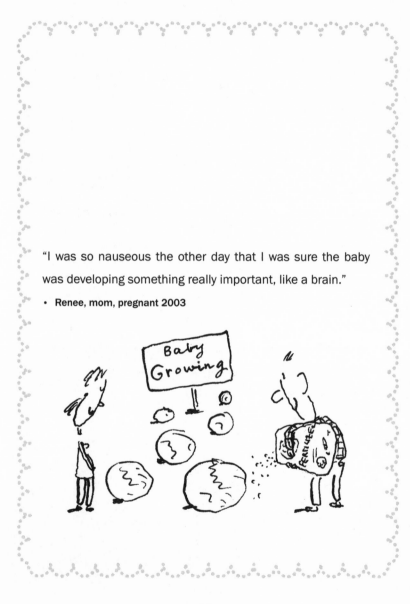

"I was so nauseous during my first few months of pregnancy that even the sight of water made me seasick, whether it was in a drinking glass or watching it on TV in *The Poseidon Adventure*."

- **Susan, waitress, pregnant 1980, 1982, 1984**

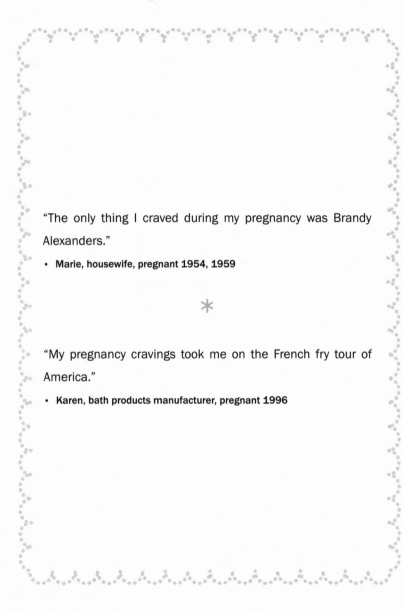

"The only thing I craved during my pregnancy was Brandy Alexanders."

- **Marie, housewife, pregnant 1954, 1959**

✳

"My pregnancy cravings took me on the French fry tour of America."

- **Karen, bath products manufacturer, pregnant 1996**

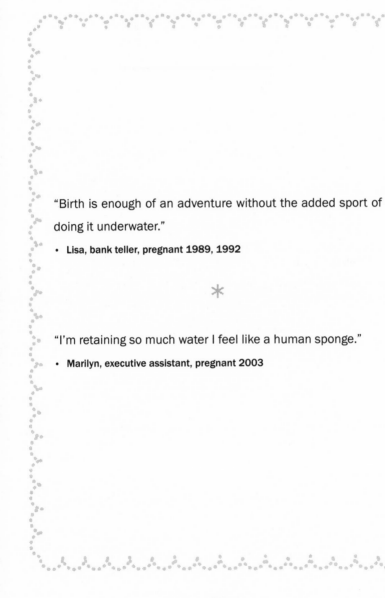

"Birth is enough of an adventure without the added sport of doing it underwater."

- **Lisa, bank teller, pregnant 1989, 1992**

✳

"I'm retaining so much water I feel like a human sponge."

- **Marilyn, executive assistant, pregnant 2003**

"Some guys are so touchy-feely with my pregnant belly that I wish they'd sprout a uterus already and experience it for themselves instead of getting their maternal fix from me."

• Julianne, media consultant, pregnant 2002

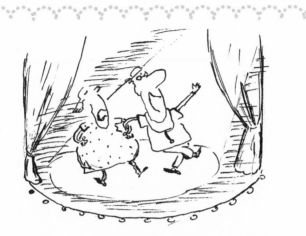

"When women smile admirably at my blooming belly I can't help but wonder if they are smiling because of the baby or because they are thinner than me."

• Alison, cashier, pregnant 2003

"As I lie here flat on my back at nine months pregnant, unable to roll over or get up without help, I imagine this is what a turtle must feel like."

- Patty, executive recruiter, pregnant 2003

"My girlfriend calls her stretch marks 'tiger claws' because of the way they look and the little cub inside who made them."

- **Liza, actress, pregnant 1990**

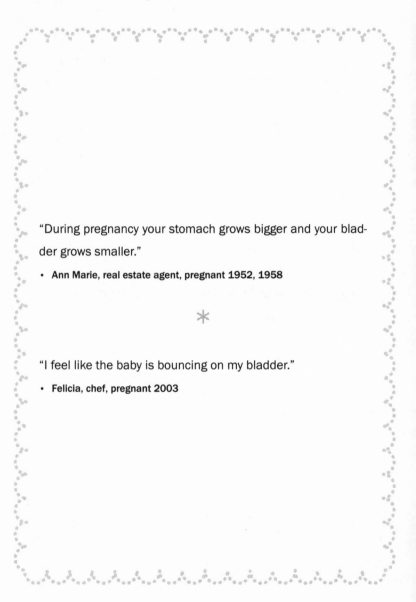

"During pregnancy your stomach grows bigger and your bladder grows smaller."

- **Ann Marie, real estate agent, pregnant 1952, 1958**

✳

"I feel like the baby is bouncing on my bladder."

- **Felicia, chef, pregnant 2003**

"My breasts were so big when I was pregnant that I felt like I was carrying three babies."

• Sue, ad copywriter, pregnant 1994, 1997, 1999

"It's a good thing that your body takes over when you're pregnant because there is no way I could make a human being—I mean, I even flunked high school biology."

• Monica, human resource manager, pregnant 1985, 1987, 1989

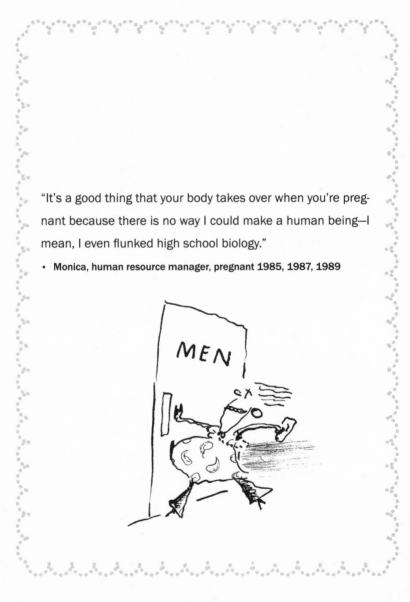

"I never knew my boss had such bad breath until I was pregnant and every little smell was intensified."

- **Teresa, real estate agent, pregnant 1997**

*

"When I was pregnant I carried around a tissue scented with my favorite perfume in my purse to put over my nose in case I ran into a smell that was undesirable."

- **Shelley, mom, pregnant 1998**

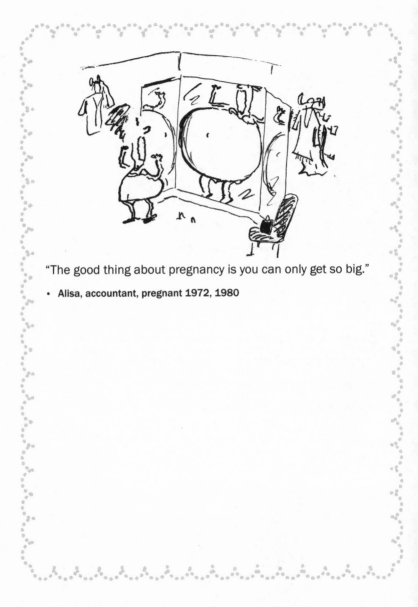

"The good thing about pregnancy is you can only get so big."

• Alisa, accountant, pregnant 1972, 1980

"One of the worst things you can say to a pregnant woman is 'What are you, nine months pregnant?' because chances are she's only five months along."

- **Miranda, director of sales and marketing, pregnant 1985, 1989**

"Sometimes it feels like the baby is using my ribs as a xylo-phone."

• Courtney, public relations specialist, pregnant 2002

✳

"Four o'clock A.M. is when my daughter wakes me up with her in utero gymnastics routine."

• Priscilla, photographer, pregnant 2003

"Having twins is like a nonstop kickboxing match going on in your belly."

• Celeste, mom, pregnant 1999, 2002

✳

"Trying to sleep when pregnant is like trying to sleep on a bag of rocks."

• Tracy, dermatologist, pregnant 1987, 1990, 1995

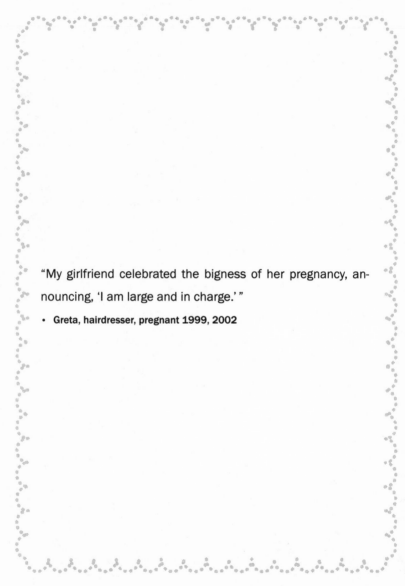

"My girlfriend celebrated the bigness of her pregnancy, announcing, 'I am large and in charge.'"

- **Greta, hairdresser, pregnant 1999, 2002**

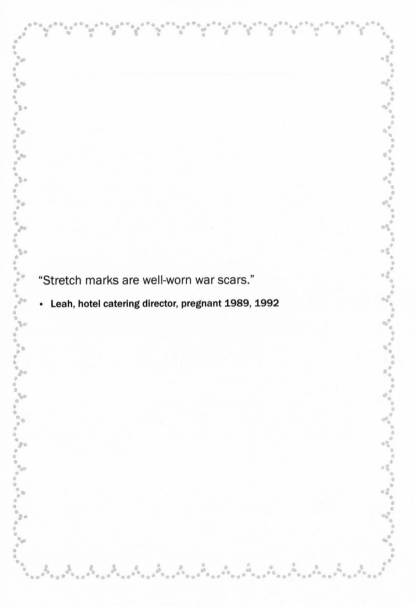

"Stretch marks are well-worn war scars."

• Leah, hotel catering director, pregnant 1989, 1992

Chapter Six

Mama Drama

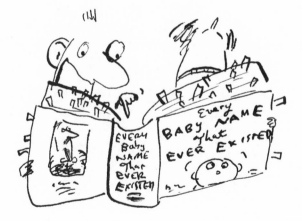

"I was sound asleep, safe in bed, when I awoke to find myself upside down and headed to the floor. My unborn son had kicked me out of bed."

• **Rose, choir director, pregnant 1960, 1962, 1963, 1970**

"I saw a very pregnant woman in the bathroom at a department store and thought, 'Man is she big. She must be due next week.' Then I caught a glimpse of myself in the mirror, and I was just as big at six months of pregnancy."

- **Ellen, high school teacher, pregnant 1996, 1998**

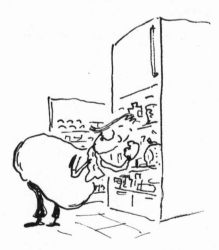

"When I was fully expanded (thirty-seven–plus weeks) with Josie in February of '99, I was lurching my way down some icy subway stairs at 23rd and Broadway and naturally slipped and fell. I was unhurt, of course, because I landed and slid down on my very ample backside. Midfall, I enjoyed the sight of a rake-thin, NYC *Sex in the City* type at the foot of the stairs: Her face a mask of fear, she darted sideways and ducked out of my way. I was tempted to ask if *she* was okay when I hoisted myself back onto my feet."

- **Annie, boxing commentator, pregnant 1999, 2002**

"My baby brother, who is not so little at thirty-two years of age, is a great uncle and loves babies but is not so keen on the whole pregnancy process. Conversations of lactation and the cuts and snips required to tidy up after birth send him wincing out of the room. As a practical joke, I asked him to videotape the impending birth of our second child, appealing to him as my favorite brother with whom I wanted to share this miraculous experience. Both honored and horrified at the same time, he agreed. We had him going right up until I was ready to push and then let him off the hook. By the relieved look on his face you would have thought he had just birthed a baby."

• Laura, actuary, pregnant 1997, 2002

"At first I wanted nine boys—enough for a baseball team. Then I had my son naturally and he's an only child."

- **Cheryl, deli lady, pregnant 1952**

✳

"So many of my friends seem to change into what they think a mother should be when they have a baby. I hope I don't lose my personality along with my placenta in the labor room."

- **Caroline, computer programmer, pregnant 2003**

"It drives me nuts when people say, 'You're actually pregnant for ten months!' because forty weeks divided by four weeks equals ten months. Have these people ever looked at a calendar? A month is about four and a half weeks, so let's keep it at the nine months it's always been and stop trying to stretch it out longer than it already is!"

• Adrian, marriage counselor, pregnant 1993, 1996

"One of the weirdest cravings I've ever heard of was told to me by my Swiss friend, who said that when his mom was pregnant she craved the smell of gas fumes and would hang out at gas pumps to satisfy her bizarre desire. He was kind of an odd guy. It made sense."

• Colleen, art director, pregnant 1997

"Choosing the right name for your newborn baby is not as easy as one would think. And one always has to be aware of the consequences—like silly nicknames or initials that spell something rude. My husband and I hadn't picked a name before the arrival of our second son, but after some debate, we agreed on Mackenzie—a suitably strong, masculine name for our robust child. It wasn't until we pulled up to our home with our new bundle of joy that we realized we had named him after the corner street where we lived. My husband exclaimed it was a good thing we didn't live on the next street over or Mackenzie would have been saddled with the most unsuitable name of Blanche!"

• Tara, president of a family-owned steel fabricating plant, pregnant 1995, 1998

"I swear this pregnancy is making me senile. The other day I was at home trying to call my husband on his cell phone and kept getting a busy signal. Then I realized I was dialing my home number over and over again. Of course it was busy . . . I was on the phone."

• Johanna, writer, pregnant 2002

✳

"Pregnancy has this way of freeing your mind. Sometimes it's a good thing, like when you're worried about how many cookies you ate the night before, and sometimes it's a bad thing, like when you forgot where you parked your car at the mall."

• Danielle, model, pregnant 1999, 2003

"Remember those Bobo doll toys, an inflatable clown weighted at the bottom that you punch and it springs back to you? That's what it feels like being pregnant, slightly off balance, and constantly being punched and kicked from a little baby inside you."

• Lucy, elementary school principal, pregnant 1975, 1978

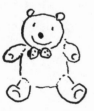

"There are days when the baby feels so heavy I think she's going to drop right out of me. And then I remember how hard I had to push with my son, and I know that baby's not coming out until I say so!"

- **Betty, human resource director, pregnant 1997, 2003**

"There's something about pregnancy that gives you the nerve to say things you normally wouldn't. My boss is a gastro-internist and has horrible hygiene. It's one thing for us in the office to suffer through his foul breath and body odor, but his poor patients! So finally I spoke up, as I was pregnant, with all my senses superheightened, and I simply couldn't stand the stench. 'It's me or the stink,' I told him in the nicest way possible. I think this 'courage to speak your mind' thing that happens is sort of a survival mode that kicks in, preparing you for motherhood. Let's face it, as a mom you have to defend your young against the world and all the nasty little smells it throws at you."

• Erin, nurse, pregnant 2001

"I had the strangest craving when I was pregnant. When I was in elementary school (circa 1970), teachers made copies of tests and paperwork using the blue ink ditto machines. I used to love the smell of the freshly printed paper and, for some bizarre reason, really wanted to experience it again. So I started calling schools and print shops looking for the old mimeograph machine and finally found it an hour outside of town. Needless to say, I drove there and got my fix."

• Heidi, telemarketer, pregnant 1986, 1988

"I've always thought the phrase 'barefoot and pregnant' was somewhat derogatory, if not downright sexist. But now that I am eight months pregnant with huge bloated duck feet, I wish I could use those words to my advantage. Like when stores and restaurants post signs that say 'Shirts and Shoes Required'... I think they should make an exception for expectant women and add: ... 'Unless You're Pregnant and None of Your Shoes Fit.' "

• Liz, financial analyst, pregnant 1992, 1995

"Forget the fact that my feet have puffed up like giant marsh-mallows; I can barely reach them over my pregnant stomach to put shoes on. One day I was late to work and rushing to get out of the house. I keep my two pairs of comfortable work shoes at the foot of my bed for easy access. As usual, I slipped on my shoes and went to work. When I got there, I noticed a lot of people staring at my feet and snickering. I had no idea what everyone was laughing about because I hadn't seen my feet in weeks. Finally my friend complimented me on my daring fashion sense, pointing out that I was wearing a cream-colored shoe on one foot and a black shoe on the other."

- **Camille, vice president of sales and marketing, pregnant 2003**

"Now that I'm pregnant I haven't been so obsessed about my choice of underwear since my wedding. Back then I was on the hunt for a sexy bra that made me look busty in and out of my wedding gown and some knockout unmentionables for our honeymoon. Now that I'm pregnant the bra is all about support and serious holster action to try and tame the ever-growing 'beasts,' as these unrecognizable things certainly aren't the 'breasts' I've come to know and love. And as for undies, I've abandoned my bikini briefs for granny panties."

• Lori, waitress, pregnant 2002

"At seven months pregnant I can barely bend over. I tried to put my underwear on today and it shot across the floor like a slingshot."

- Robin, landscape architect, pregnant 2003

✳

"At first, you're trying to get pregnant and you're a slave to the tick-tock of your biological clock. Then you get pregnant and you're a slave to the drip-drop on the clock of the pregnant woman's bladder."

- Vanessa, flight attendant, pregnant 1990

"I had spent thirty-four years of my life trying not to get pregnant. Then my husband and I made the happy decision to 'go for it.' But when I saw those two lines on the pregnancy stick I freaked. My husband kept saying, 'Are you all right? You're as white as a ghost. You look like you're going to faint.' Of course, later that day I was ecstatic, but my initial reaction was as if I was sixteen years old, thinking, 'I am going to be in so much trouble with my parents.'"

· Jill, corporate planner, pregnant 2001

"My sister is a real prankster and she got me good when I was nine months pregnant. We were shopping for groceries together when all of a sudden she said she had left the tea-kettle on at home and needed to go outside to call the neighbor to go into her house and turn it off. Anyway, I was in the checkout line when the manager came up to me and discreetly asked me to go with him. I asked if there was a problem and he said, 'There won't be if you come quietly.' I had no idea what was going on. When we were behind closed doors he said that someone had seen me slip a watermelon under my shirt. I told him that I was pregnant with a baby, not a melon. He said that they had seen this ploy before and would I kindly prove it. I lifted my shirt just enough for him to turn beet red and start apologizing profusely. He gave me the groceries for free and I found my sister out by the car laughing her head off."

- Jackie, administrative assistant, pregnant 1982, 1987

"With the second pregnancy, your body reacts like an old pair of jeans. They may be nice and tight out of the wash, holding in every little bulge, but wear them for a day and they expand to fit your size, whatever it may be."

- Marissa, mom, pregnant 1998, 2001

"I was shocked at how the human body remembers its pregnant state the second time around. It's as if it has a 'been there, done that' mentality that forces you to get with the program emotionally. I kept feeling like, 'Wait, slow down. I'm only three months pregnant so why do I look like I am six months along?' It was a little too quick for me, leaving my head to play catch-up each month."

• Catherine, pharmaceutical sales rep, pregnant 1999, 2003

"My stretch marks look like funky rays of light coming out of my belly button. My own personal sun! Pretty cool."

• Jacqui, stay-at-home mom, pregnant 1997, 1998, 2000

✳

"I was never 'baby drunk'—you know, those women who get all loopy at the sight of an infant. In fact, as a teen, I secretly feared that the doctors would tell me that I was too little to have babies. I'm only 4'11"! But then I realized babies are only about twenty inches when they come out and they really are cute."

• Anne, legal assistant, pregnant 2002

Chapter Seven

Father Time

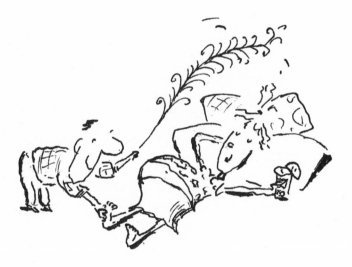

"I learned early on when my wife complained about the weight she was gaining to simply listen and then say, 'Baby, you're not fat, you're pregnant.'"

• **Tom, bank executive, wife pregnant 1985, 1988**

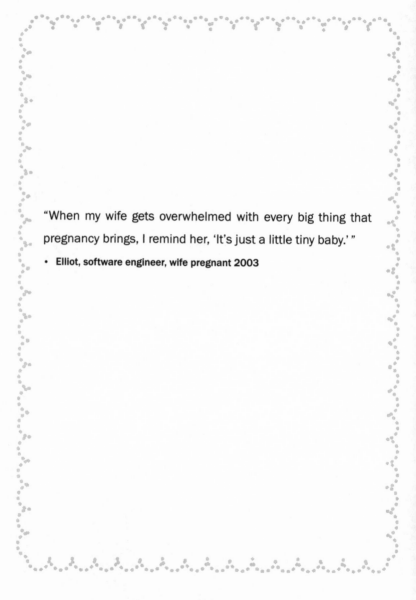

"When my wife gets overwhelmed with every big thing that pregnancy brings, I remind her, 'It's just a little tiny baby.' "

• **Elliot, software engineer, wife pregnant 2003**

"I was six months pregnant and we decided to take a vacation in Hawaii. I had worked out during my entire pregnancy and felt perfectly comfortable wearing my new red bikini. When watching the video that my husband took during the vacation, I saw myself in the red bikini from behind and thought, 'Damn, my butt looks great for being six months pregnant!' Then the woman in the red bikini turned around and it wasn't me."

- Lizzie, nurse, pregnant 1998, 2003

"Our male friends are envious of my husband, thinking that he's reaping the benefits of the natural breast enhancement that occurs with pregnancy. What they don't understand is that it's a 'look, don't touch' situation, as they're so tender that I'd be in pain if he went near them and then I'd have to inflict pain upon him."

- **Alexandra, pharmacist, pregnant 2002**

"My husband, being a devout breast man, views my enlarged pregnant bosom as a sort of anatomical Disneyland."

- Frances, plumber, pregnant 1999, 2003

"My wife went into labor at the beauty salon while having her highlights done. But instead of rinsing and heading to the hospital, she insisted they finish the job, as she knew many would be taking her picture after the baby was born."

• Ken, attorney, wife pregnant 1982, 1984, 1986

✳

"I adore my wife, but 'whine and dine' has a whole new meaning when you take your pregnant spouse out to dinner."

• Allan, civil engineer, wife pregnant 1999, 2003

"We were traveling back from Australia with a stopover in Los Angeles and decided to get a snack in one of those sundries stores. My wife spied a spicy Cajun pepper beef jerky stick and said to me, 'Wow, that looks good.' I turned to her, a quizzical look on my face (as she doesn't like jerky) and said, 'You're pregnant.' I was right."

- Jonathon, movie producer, wife pregnant 1995

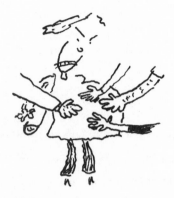

"My husband affectionately called me 'Frankenstein feet' during my pregnancy because my feet had become so swollen that they looked like the big foot blocks on the monster."

• **Kristina, mom, pregnant 1990, 1994**

"I've always said that my wife is the ultimate trooper. I was in a remote part of Mexico on business a month before my wife's due date and got into a bad car accident. My darling wife hopped on a plane and rushed to my side. After a couple of weeks in the hospital the doctor said I could go home, but when we got to the airport it was another story. They wouldn't let my wife on the airplane because she was due in a week and they couldn't take the risk. Fortunately we had taken Lamaze and were planning a natural childbirth, so we felt in control of the situation as opposed to relying on my broken Spanish to request pain medication or anything else. When the time came we went back to the hospital and my wife gave birth to our beautiful daughter—no epidural was administered and no English was spoken. We went home a week later with our baby and a birth certificate that says something in Spanish."

- **Gerry, importer, wife pregnant 1990, 1993**

"My wife and I disagreed about many birthing issues. We were both for natural childbirth, but she wanted to stay at home and do it in the bathtub and I wanted us to be in a hospital in case anything went wrong. We actually sat down and negotiated a labor contract."

• Patrick, music executive, wife pregnant 2002

"My wife and I were devout hippies in the 1960s. She gave birth to our son at home, where I delivered him, and I've been getting him out of tight situations ever since."

- **Carl, teacher, wife pregnant 1964, 1967**

"My wife and I are avid basketball fans, and she wasn't about to let a little condition like pregnancy keep us from floor seats at the NBA playoffs. She had to use the bathroom since the beginning of the second period but couldn't tear herself away from the game. The second the buzzer sounded at halftime we bolted to the bathroom, only to find the line for the ladies' room a mile long. There was no way she could wait and I had a feeling that this competitive crowd of women wouldn't tolerate cutting in line, especially when a few of them were pregnant as well. She grabbed my arm and headed for the men's room. 'Cover me,' she said and boldly marched into the guys' side. 'Pregnant lady coming through!' she announced. 'Don't worry, guys. Obviously there's nothing I haven't seen before.' I stood guard outside the stall until she was done, and no one said a word. She's a smart one, knowing that no man would deny a gutsy pregnant woman."

- **Rick, tax attorney, wife pregnant 1999**

"My husband and I have always had silly nicknames for each other. During pregnancy I awoke most mornings to 'Good morning, Preg Nancy.' When I would try and figure something out, like where I put the keys, he would say, 'Solve the mystery yet, Preg Nancy Drew?' While singing along with the radio, I got 'Sounds good, Preg Nancy Sinatra.' And when the baby was in a punchy mood we would watch my belly for entertainment, and he called that *The Preg Nancy and Sluggo Show.* My husband's such a nut."

• **Annabelle, architect, pregnant 1995, 2000**

"My husband and I have a deal. I carry the baby for nine months and he changes diapers for the nine months after that. I think it's fair."

• Judy, customer service rep, pregnant 2002

✳

"The other day my husband said, 'Wow, it seems like this pregnancy is going a lot quicker than the last one.' I wanted to punch him."

• Danielle, restaurant hostess, pregnant 2000

"My wife had a bit of performance anxiety about the birth of our child. She wanted to go natural, as many of her friends had, and didn't even want to consider wimping out with an epidural. She kept bringing up how the previous summer when we went hiking she'd barely made it to the top of the mountain and on the way down I had to carry her backpack because she was so tired. I tried to reassure her, saying, 'Well, you're not really the outdoorsy, mountain-climbing type, honey. But I've seen how you attack the sweater pile in a department store sale. You always hang in there until you get what you want.' During her labor she whispered to me, 'I'm visualizing myself at Macy's in a crowd of ferocious shoppers swarming around a table of cashmere sweaters.' Sure enough, she had our new baby girl without the use of any drugs. As a gift I gave both mama and baby very expensive cashmere sweaters."

• Jason, film editor, wife pregnant 2000

"After eight months of a moody pregnancy, my husband said, 'I want my wife back,' to which I responded, 'I want that woman back, too, but I'll settle for just her butt.'"

- Raye, producer, pregnant 1998, 2002

*

"My husband was so relaxed that he fell asleep in Lamaze."

- Jesse, court reporter, pregnant 1997

"My husband is in naturally great shape. The other night he announced that he might start working out to sculpt his abdomen into more of a 'cut' look. As I lay there in bed seven months pregnant with my 'domed' look, I said, 'Don't you dare. There is no way you're going to look fabulous when I have to look like this. We're in this together through thick and thin.' He apologized and ate his ice cream sundae."

- **Erica, shipping manager, pregnant 2003**

"Even with the epidural, my wife was in excruciating pain giving birth to our ten-pound son. I felt like I needed an epidural just listening to her."

• Ed, IT operations manager, wife pregnant 1997, 1999

"They should offer husbands a little medication or at least set up a bar behind the nurses' station in the labor ward to take the edge off what you just saw your wife go through and what you just saw go through her."

• James, chief financial officer, wife pregnant 1998, 2002

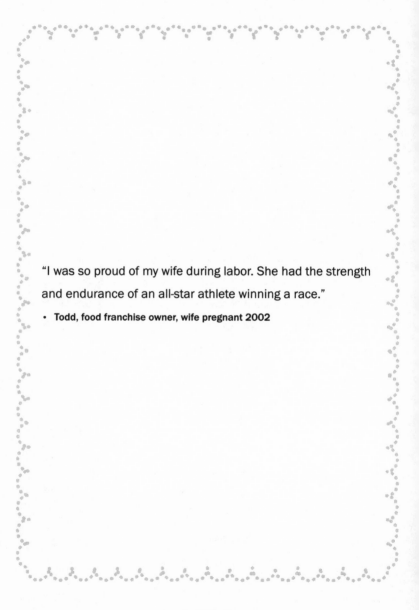

"I was so proud of my wife during labor. She had the strength and endurance of an all-star athlete winning a race."

• **Todd, food franchise owner, wife pregnant 2002**

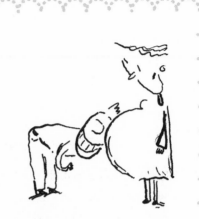

"As my wife was in labor pushing, I found myself pushing along with her. It was such a workout that afterward I felt the 'burn' in my abs."

- **Kellan, graphic artist, wife pregnant 2003**

"My husband wanted his 'mommy' in the labor room with us when I gave birth. There was no way that was going to happen, but I tried to respect his feelings. Besides the fact that I knew I'd be in pain and cursing like a sailor, which would totally offend her, I wasn't crazy about her seeing my 'girly parts,' a sight that my own mother hasn't seen in a very long time. After my initial shock wore off I calmly said, 'Well, she wasn't there when we conceived the child and she won't be there to see me push it out of my body.' "

• **Kathleen, creative director, pregnant 2003**

Chapter Eight

Stay Out of My Womb!

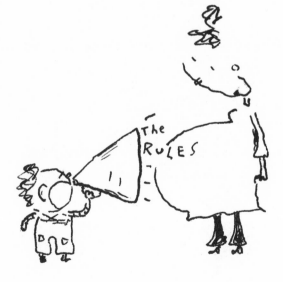

"My little girl wouldn't let me have bubble gum when I was pregnant for fear that I would swallow it and blow up the baby."

- **Shelby, nursery school teacher, pregnant 1989**

＊

" 'Mommy, is your tummy going to explode?' asked my five-year-old son when I was eight months pregnant."

- **John's mommy, pregnant 1985, 1989**

"My four-year-old son thought the baby was in one of my breasts rather than my belly because they had grown so big."

• Kevin's mommy, pregnant 1998, 2002

∗

"When my belly button popped out, as most pregnant women's belly buttons do, my little boy told me, 'Don't worry, Mommy, it's just the baby's finger poking it.' "

• Evan's mommy, pregnant 1986, 1990

"The whole family was present for the twenty-week structural ultrasound of the baby. One would think that the conversation would be all about the baby's development, but with our five-year-old son in the room it became all about him. After singing three rounds of the *Scooby-Doo* theme song, he announced that he saw a chicken in my tummy playing with the baby. He said he saw the beak and feathers, which were actually the baby's nose and fingers. Later in the examining room, he told the doctor to be sure and get the chicken out when he was removing the baby."

- **Dylan's mommy, pregnant 1998, 2003**

"My little boy came with us for a doctor's appointment and was thrilled to hear the baby's heartbeat through the Doppler. When we got home, he wanted to hear it again by any means possible. When his play stethoscope didn't work, he tried hooking me up to this superspy hearing device, which is like a toy surveillance gadget with headphones and a mini satellite dish that magnifies sound. It didn't really work well either, so he just put his ear to my belly and was satisfied with that."

- Brandon's mommy, pregnant 1989, 2002

"When we found out that we were expecting, we explained to our six-year-old girl all the things that were going to happen, such as, 'Mommy's tummy is going to grow because that is where the baby will be.' When I was seven months pregnant, our daughter said, 'Mommy, I'm confused.' Thinking that she needed to share her feelings about the new baby, I said, 'What's the matter, dear?' She replied, 'Well, if the baby is only growing in your tummy, how come your butt is getting so big?'"

- **Courtney's mommy, pregnant 1992, 1998, 2001**

"At around twenty-five weeks of pregnancy, most every woman has to drink this orange soda concoction in order to take her glucose test. Well, we don't have juice, let alone any kind of artificial colored soda, in the house, and when my son saw me drinking it he screamed, 'Mama, stop!' I asked him, 'What's wrong?' He said, 'If you drink that, the baby will turn orange like a pumpkin!' "

- Charlie's mommy, pregnant 1999, 2003

" 'Mama, the baby's knocking. Let her out!' is what my three-year-old daughter said when she saw the impression of the baby's fist punching from inside my pregnant belly."

• Chloe's mommy, pregnant 1995, 2000

"We encouraged our little son to talk to the baby in the womb. He said, 'Can the baby really hear me?' 'Yes,' we replied, thinking he was going to vow his big-brotherly love to her. 'Good, because I have something important to say.' And he proceeded to lay down the ground rules: 'There are some toys you can play with but other ones you can't, and if you chew on anything I'm going to chew on you, but just pretend chewing.' "

• **Skyler's mommy, pregnant 1988, 1991**

"Our daughter loved talking to the baby in the womb. She gave him the lowdown on us as parents, saying, 'Mama is really nice and smells pretty, but she makes me clean up my room. Daddy always has a scratchy face, but you can see far away when you sit on his shoulders.'"

• Hannah's mommy, pregnant 1998, 2001

"My little boy overheard me say 'I have a bun in the oven' while patting my pregnant belly. A couple of days later I was making hamburgers and asked him to get the buns out of the pantry and he said, 'Let's just use the bun that's in your tummy oven, Mommy.' "

- Jarod's mommy, pregnant 2001, 2003

"We sat down our two-year-old and explained that Mommy has a baby in her belly. Much to our relief he was really excited. You never know how a little guy is going to react to sharing his mommy. The next day he said, 'Mommy, do you have bacon in your belly?' I cracked up, not really knowing what he meant, and clarified, 'No, it's a real baby boy just like you. What shall we name him?' 'Bacon,' he said, as if this had been his point all along and I was just starting to catch on. Now my husband and I joke that 'Mom's makin' Bacon.' "

• Reese's mommy, pregnant 2000, 2003

"I was so thrilled that our four-year-old son wanted to participate in all aspects of my pregnancy with his little brother. He even came with me to every doctor's appointment. On one occasion, the doctor expressed concern about my weight gain, as I had put on about fifty pounds. The doctor tried to couch his concern by addressing my son, saying, 'Has Mommy been eating a lot of candy?' And my son replied, 'No, but she's been eating a whole lot of cookies and brownies.'"

- **Miles's mommy, pregnant 1998, 2002**

"Mommy, when you rub your tummy the baby will come out of your belly button like a genie."

- Davey, mommy pregnant 2001, 2003

✳

"We discovered that I had developed gestational diabetes in my thirtieth week of pregnancy. We explained to our five-year-old son that Mommy was no longer eating any dessert because the sugar wasn't good for the baby. Our son said, 'That's okay, Mommy. When you want a cookie just kiss me. I'm sweet enough for both of us.'"

- Tommy's mommy, pregnant 1998, 2003

Chapter Nine

Labor of Love

Yoo hoo

"My wife's water broke in the town car en route to the hospital. When we arrived, someone on the bottom floor told us
about a quicker way to get up to the maternity ward. We got
lost and my wife said, 'I feel the baby coming.' On the freight
elevator she said, 'I feel the head!' When we finally got to the
correct floor I was sure I heard screaming from inside her
sweatpants."

• **Michael, investor relations executive, wife pregnant 2003**

"I went into labor at four A.M. on the morning of the Los Angeles Gay Pride Parade and the only day that the main street to the hospital would be blocked off. When we arrived, my contractions had slowed down considerably, and the staff suggested that I go home and wait it out. We considered our options: stay at the hospital and probably be induced, or go home and try to make our way back in the middle of the parade with the chance that our baby could be delivered by a team of Marilyn Monroe drag queens on the back of a float."

• Linda, ad executive, pregnant 1999

"I'd seen it so often on TV and in movies that I thought the only way to know the baby was coming was if your water broke. When I found out the truth, I spent weeks worrying over whether or not I'd actually know when I went into labor. But when it came time, believe me, I knew!"

• Briana, marketing director, pregnant 2000

✳

"I was flat on my back when my water broke, and it shot up like a geyser. It looked like Old Faithful coming over a mountain."

• Pamela, boutique owner, pregnant 1961, 1962, 1965

"My sister had been in labor for sixteen hours without any epidural (overachiever!). Finally she was dilated to ten, and the doctor told Gina that it was time to push. Gina looked over at me and said, 'Hand me my pants!' Of course I was shocked and asked her what she wanted her pants for. She said, 'Because I am going home. *I am not doing this anymore!'* My brother-in-law and I started laughing, as we thought that Linda Blair had taken over her body, and then she started yelling, 'YOU DON'T UNDERSTAND, NONE OF YOU UNDERSTAND!!!!' This little voice from the corner of the hospital room said, 'I do. Now pull yourself together and push that baby out!' It was our mom, who, obviously, had been through labor twice. I guess that is what my sister needed because she calmed down and got to business and delivered a beautiful baby girl forty minutes later!"

• Angie's sister, Gina, housewife, pregnant 1994, 1999

"Much to my horror, my water broke in the middle of the grocery store. Thinking fast, I threw a bottle of apple juice on the floor to camouflage the situation."

• **Kelly, baker, pregnant 1995**

✳

"I was well into my labor contractions, and feeling no pain thanks to the epidural, when all of a sudden my water broke. It was such a warm, soothing sensation, like a wave of comfort washing over me. It felt great."

• **Sharon, interior designer, pregnant 1989, 1992**

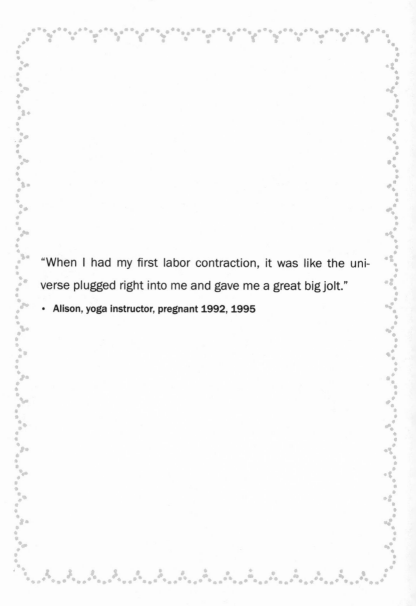

"When I had my first labor contraction, it was like the universe plugged right into me and gave me a great big jolt."

• Alison, yoga instructor, pregnant 1992, 1995

"During my au natural labor, my husband gently cupped my shoulders, faced me, and said, 'Baby, just try and relax.' I dug my claws into his shoulders and said, 'There! How does that feel? Now you try and relax, baby!' "

- **Raye, producer, pregnant 1998, 2002**

"My family has always been competitive. There I was in a Los Angeles hospital room, doubled over with painful labor contractions, when my brother, sister, and father called me on the cell phone from a New York City bar, supposedly to check up on me. What I later found out is that they had a betting pool going on the baby's time of birth."

• **Kate, office manager, pregnant 2001**

"I heard of all these wacky ideas that are supposed to bring on labor. Drinking raspberry vinegar, bouncing vigorously on a bouncy ball, and the oddest is downing a dose of castor oil. Is the oil going to make the baby simply slide out of you? What worked for me in the beginning and in the end was having sex. One good climax and my uterus was contracting like a builder after an earthquake."

- **Bonnie, professional dog walker, pregnant 2000**

"My wife had been in labor, pushing, for thirty-five hours, refusing any pain medication. She made me swear not to let anyone give her anything or, as she put it, 'You will never live it down for the rest of your life.' Well, her family was getting restless and started pressuring me to get her an epidural because they couldn't stand to see her suffer. Finally the doctor decided to break her water, which would speed up labor and make the contractions even more painful. With this info the family really ganged up on me to urge her to take something for the pain. So I privately asked the doctor, 'How much longer before the baby comes out?' He said, 'Usually about six hours.' I went back to the family and said, 'The doctor thinks it's only going to be another two hours. We're almost there and she really wants to go natural.' The family relaxed a bit and by some miracle the baby was born an hour and a half later."

- Ethan, engineer, wife pregnant 2001

"I was four weeks past my due date and finally went into labor on a Thursday. By Friday afternoon I had progressed a bit, but held off on the epidural as I had heard that it could slow down the labor process and this baby did not want to come out! Late Friday night all signs were good and I was pretty uncomfortable. At the stroke of midnight, I couldn't stand the pain any longer and requested an epidural. The anesthesiologist came into the room all bright and cheery, given the wee hour, and announced, 'It's my birthday!' She gave me the epidural and an hour later my son was born. Shortly afterward she popped into my hospital room and said to the baby, 'Since it's both of our birthdays tell your mommy that the epidural is on me,' and she didn't charge me for it."

• **Effie, gourmet caterer, pregnant 1997**

Chapter Ten

Heartwarmers

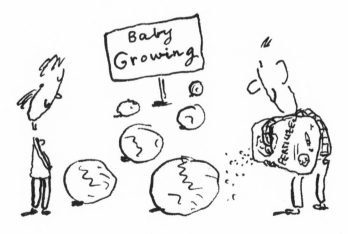

"I know what the baby feels like on the inside; I just don't know what the baby is going to feel like on the outside."

- **Justine, actress, pregnant 2000**

" 'I can't wait until this is over,' I said to my mother as I patted my nine-months-pregnant belly. 'Oh dear,' my mother chuckled, 'it's never over. Not when the baby is out of you, not when your baby's all grown up, and especially not when your baby's having a baby.' "

• **Holly, ceramics teacher, pregnant 1992**

"My fingers had swelled so much during my pregnancy that I had to take off my wedding ring. I was heartbroken. I hadn't removed the ring since my husband placed it there on our wedding day. But I had heard stories about women who had to have their rings cut off their fat pregnant fingers and I would have sooner cut off my finger than destroy the ring. A friend suggested that I wear it around my neck on a chain right next to my heart. I loved this idea! As we approached the baby's due date my husband wanted me to take the ring necklace off and put it in a safe place in our home. He didn't want me to go into labor somewhere and have something that valuable in our hospital room. I said we'd have plenty of time because we had to get the suitcase at home anyway. We got into a big fight that ended with me ripping the chain off my neck and tossing it in the jewelry box. A week later our beautiful baby girl was born and my husband surprised me with a brand-new diamond in my wedding ring."

- **Cathleen, insurance claims adjuster, pregnant 2003**

"Thing is, for every three 'negative' New York maternity experiences, there's always one gem to offset them, like a cab-driver who refused to accept my money because I was with child."

- **Anne, writer, pregnant 1999, 2002**

＊

"A mother's child is the virtuoso of her heartstrings."

- **Simone, composer, pregnant 1998, 2003**

"I recently learned from *American Baby* that 71 percent of first-time mothers find out the sex of their baby. I decided not to be a part of that majority. One reason was that a friend and recent mom told me that the only thing that got her through her very tough last six weeks was not knowing. She felt she could wait it out because at the end she would get to know the gender. I bought into that approach. Five weeks and counting, and all I want to do is meet this little boy or girl."

- **Lauren, book packager, pregnant 2003**

"I affectionately call our little boy 'a sucker baby.' He's so pre-cious he sucks you into having another one immediately."

- **Debbie, casting director, pregnant 1998, 2000**

"Everyone looks at me with a combination of pity and horror when they find out I am expecting twins, but I feel like the luckiest woman alive. I have twice as much love inside me!"

• Sylvie, wine shop owner, pregnant 2003

"It's funny how you can predict the personality of the baby in the womb. My five-year-old son has been a persistent little guy right from the start. When I was pregnant with him he didn't like it when I lay on my side and would rhythmically kick me until I rolled over onto my back. To this day he'll fight to the end to get what he wants, and it's one of the qualities I love most in him!"

• Marcia, illustrator, pregnant 1998

"When we found out we were pregnant with our first child, a boy, thoughts of his childhood came to mind—skinned knees, baseball, and creepy-crawly things. When we found out that the second child we were expecting was a girl, our thoughts raced ahead to her teen and adult years—the prom, marriage, and a baby of her own."

- **Kendra, accounting assistant, pregnant 1994, 1997**

"After I had given birth, my husband went with the baby to the nursery for his first bath, and I went to my hospital room accompanied by my brother and mother. My husband returned proudly wheeling in the bassinet with our new little son, Dylan. Next to the baby in the bassinet was a black velvet jewelry box. My husband said, 'Dylan and I have a gift for you.' Inside the box was a pair of gorgeous pearl earrings, as pearl was the baby's birthstone. Everyone's eyes welled up and I was so happy that we had a boy because the world could use more men as wonderful as his father."

• Jeanne, author, pregnant 1998, 2003

"My relationship with my mother has always been a little strained. I never knew why—if it was because we were too similar, too different, who knows? I had gone into labor on a Friday morning and, in between contractions, made all the calls to family members, letting them know that our baby was on her way. By Friday evening I was still walking the hospital hallways, contracting a lot, not dilating much, eating ice chips, and all the business that goes with the labor process. Then down the corridor I saw my mom. She had hopped in the car right after I called her and driven from San Francisco to Los Angeles to be with me. The second I saw the look on my mother's face, a mixture of excitement, concern, bliss, help-lessness, strength . . . I got it. I understood where she was coming from. In that very moment I realized that being a mom is about a lot of things, and many of those things are going to create a strain with your child. But mostly it's about being there for your child when they need you."

• Missy, executive headhunter, pregnant 2001

"We had just bought a new home and, unbeknownst to me, I was five weeks pregnant. I hadn't been feeling quite right so I took the pregnancy test one afternoon and, yep, I was expecting. My husband and I had been so busy with the move that we were very casual about the whole baby thing. Well, I wanted to call him immediately, but then I had a better idea. I went to the grocery store and bought ten cabbages. I also picked up a little white picket sign. After lining up the cabbages in a remote part of the backyard, I wrote Baby Growing on the sign and stuck it right smack in the middle of the patch. When my husband came home from work I said, 'Honey! We have a cabbage patch in the yard.' 'Oh, great,' he said, 'now we're going to attract rabbits, moles, and every other creature looking for dinner.' I still had to get him out there so I said, 'You know, I think I did see a bunny.' He raced outside, with me fast on his heels, and stopped short at the cabbage patch. He turned to me with a smirk, gave me a big kiss, and said, 'You're going to be a really fun mom.'"

- **Rhonda, travel agent, pregnant 2003**

"I love it when midwives call themselves 'baby catchers.' It makes childbirth sound so easy, so safe, and so natural."

• **Bridget, nurse, pregnant 1986, 1988**

"I love it when the baby hiccups in the womb. The feeling of being pregnant can be so alien, and something as simple as a hiccup feels so familiar."

- **Susan, makeup sales rep, pregnant 2002**

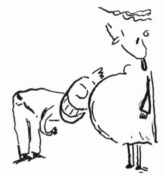

"I'm not really the 'gooey' type. I don't cry at sappy movies and I don't coo at babies, although I think they're pretty cool. I didn't even cry when my baby was born, which worried me a bit. 'What kind of mother will I be?' I asked my husband, completely dry-eyed, after he put our precious newborn in my arms. 'You'll be yourself,' he said, knowing I'm not one for manufacturing emotion, no matter what the circumstances. Later that evening, my family came to the hospital to see the baby. My dad tried to seize a photo op with my mother by my bedside and my grandmother holding the baby. Then it hit me. This is a life that we've created, a future full of hopes and dreams and many more generations to come. Well, my dad never took the photo because I was bawling my eyes out."

• Joan, film editor, pregnant 2000

About the Author

Jeanne Benedict balances her career as a TV host and author of three books on entertaining and cooking with being an adoring mommy. Known as a chef and designer, she has styled everything from lavish parties to home décor. She lives in Los Angeles with her family, and at the time of this publication she will have been pregnant for 1.5 years.